MIGRAINE And Other HEADACHES

The most common type of headache is a tension headache. Tension headaches are due to tight muscles in your shoulders, neck, scalp and jaw. They are often related to stress, depression or anxiety. You are more likely to get tension headaches if you work too much, don't get enough sleep, miss meals or use alcohol.

Other common types of headaches include migraines, cluster headaches and sinus headaches. Most people can feel much better by making lifestyle changes, learning ways to relax and taking pain relievers.

Headaches can have many causes, but serious causes of headaches are rare. Sometimes headaches warn of a more serious disorder. Let your health care provider know if you have sudden, severe headaches.

Get medical help right away if you have a headache after a blow to your head, or if you have a headache along with a stiff neck, fever, confusion, loss of consciousness or pain in the eye or ear.

MIGRAINE

A migraine is a common type of headache that may occur with symptoms such as nausea, vomiting, or sensitivity to light. In many people, a throbbing pain is felt only on one side of the head.

Some people who get migraines have warning symptoms, called an aura, before the actual headache begins. An aura is a group of symptoms, usually vision disturbances that serve as a warning sign that a bad headache is coming. Most people, however, do not have such warning signs.

Causes

A lot of people get migraines -- about 11 out of 100. The headaches tend to first appear between the ages of 10 and 46. Occasionally, migraines may occur later in life in a person with no history of such headaches. Migraines occur more often in women than men, and may run in families. Women may have fewer migraines when they are pregnant. Most women with such headaches have fewer attacks during the last two trimesters of pregnancy.

A migraine is caused by abnormal brain activity, which is triggered by stress, certain foods, environmental factors, or something else. However, the exact chain of events remains unclear.

Scientists used to believe that migraines were due to changes in blood vessels within the brain. Today, most medical experts believe the attack actually begins in the brain itself, where it involves various nerve pathways and chemicals. The changes affect blood flow in the brain and surrounding tissues.

Migraine attacks may be triggered by:

- Alcohol
- Allergic reactions
- Bright lights
- Certain odours or perfumes
- Changes in hormone levels (which can occur during a woman's menstrual cycle or   with the use of birth control pills)
- Changes in sleep patterns
- Exercise
- Loud noises
- Missed meals
- Physical or emotional stress
- Smoking or exposure to smoke

Certain foods and preservatives in foods may trigger migraines in some people. Food-related triggers may include:

- Any processed, fermented, pickled, or marinated foods
- Baked goods
- Chocolate
- Dairy products
- Foods containing monosodium glutamate (MSG)
- Foods containing tyramine, which includes red wine, aged cheese, smoked fish, chicken livers, figs, and certain beans
- Fruits (avocado, banana, citrus fruit)
- Meats containing nitrates (bacon, hot dogs, salami, cured meats)
- Nuts
- Onions

- Peanut butter

This list may not include all triggers.

True migraine headaches are not a result of a brain tumor or other serious medical problem. However, only an experienced health care provider can determine whether your symptoms are due to a migraine or another condition.

Symptoms:

Vision disturbances, or aura, are considered a "warning sign" that a migraine is coming. The aura occurs in both eyes and may involve any or all of the following:

- A temporary blind spot
- Blurred vision
- Eye pain
- Seeing stars or zigzag lines
- Tunnel vision

Not every person with migraines has an aura. Those who do usually develop one about 10 - 15 minutes before the headache. However, it may occur just a few minutes to 24 hours beforehand. A headache may not always follow an aura.

Migraine headaches can be dull or severe. The pain may be felt behind the eye or in the back of the head and neck. For many patients, the headaches start on the same side each time. The headaches usually:

- Feel throbbing, pounding, or pulsating
- Are worse on one side of the head
- Start as a dull ache and get worse within minutes to hours
- Last 6 to 48 hours

Other symptoms that may occur with the headache include:

- Chills
- Increased urination
- Fatigue
- Loss of appetite
- Nausea and vomiting

- Numbness, tingling, or weakness
- Problems concentrating, trouble finding words
- Sensitivity to light or sound
- Sweating

Symptoms may linger even after the migraine has gone away. Patients with migraine sometimes call this a migraine "hangover." Symptoms can include:

- Feeling mentally dull, like your thinking is not clear or sharp
- Increased need for sleep
- Neck pain

Tests:

Your doctor can diagnose this type of headache by asking questions about your symptoms and family history of migraines. A complete physical exam will be done to determine if your headaches are due to muscle tension, sinus problems, or a serious brain disorder.

There is no specific test to prove that your headache is actually a migraine. However, your doctor may order a brain MRI or CT scan if you have never had one before.

If you have a migraine with unusual symptoms such as weakness, memory problems, or loss of alertness, an EEG may be needed to rule out seizures. A lumbar puncture (spinal tap) might be done.

Treatment:

There is no specific cure for migraine headaches. The goal is to prevent symptoms by avoiding or changing your triggers.

A good way to identify triggers is to keep a headache diary. Write down:

- When your headaches occur
- How severe they are
- What you've eaten
- How much sleep you had
- Other symptoms
- Other possible factors (women should note where they are in their menstrual cycle)

For example, the diary may reveal that your headaches tend to occur more often on days when you wake up earlier than usual. Changing your sleep schedule may result in fewer migraine attacks.

When you do get migraine symptoms, try to treat them right away. The headache may be less severe. When migraine symptoms begin:

- Drink water to avoid dehydration, especially if you have vomited
- Rest in a quiet, darkened room
- Place a cool cloth on your head

Many different medications are available for people with migraines. Medicines are used to:

- Reduce the number of attacks
- Stop the migraine once early symptoms occur
- Treat the pain and other symptoms

REDUCING ATTACKS

If you have frequent migraines, your doctor may prescribe medicine to reduce the number of attacks. Such medicine needs to be taken every day in order to be effective.

STOPPING AN ATTACK

Other medicines are taken at the first sign of a migraine attack. Over-the-counter pain medications such as acetaminophen, ibuprofen, or aspirin are often helpful, especially when your migraine is mild. If these don't help, ask your doctor about prescription medications. (Be aware, however, that overuse or misuse of such pain medications may result in rebound headaches. Chronic rebound headaches typically occur in people who take pain medications more than 3 days a week on an ongoing basis.)

Patients who have nausea and vomiting with their migraines may be prescribed a nasal spray, suppository, or injection instead of pills.

Some migraine medicines narrow your blood vessels and should not be used if you are at risk for heart attacks or have heart disease, unless otherwise instructed by your health care provider. Ergots should not be taken if you are pregnant or planning to become pregnant, because they can cause serious side effects to an unborn baby.

TREATING SYMPTOMS

Other medications are primarily given to treat the symptoms of migraine.

Used alone or in combinations, these drugs can reduce your pain, nausea, or emotional distress.

If you wish to consider an alternative, feverfew is a popular herb for migraines. Several studies, but not all, support using feverfew for treating migraines. If you are interested in trying feverfew, make sure your doctor approves. Work with a trained herbalist when selecting herbs.

TYPES

Migraines are classified according to the symptoms they produce. The two most common types are migraine with aura and migraine without aura. Less common types include the following:

- Abdominal migraine
- Basilar artery migraine
- Carotidynia
- Headache-free migraine (aura without migraine)
- Ophthalmologic migraine/Ocular migraine
- Status migrainosus

Some women experience migraine headaches just prior to or during menstruation. These headaches, which are called menstrual migraines, may be related to hormonal changes and often do not occur or lessen during pregnancy. Other women develop migraines for the first time during pregnancy or after menopause.

Migraine with aura is characterized by a neurological phenomenon (aura) that is experienced 10 to 30 minutes before the headache. Most auras are visual and are described as bright shimmering lights around objects or at the edges of the field of vision (called scintillating scotomas) or zigzag lines, castles (teichopsia), wavy images, or hallucinations. Others experience temporary vision loss. No visual auras include motor weakness, speech or language abnormalities, dizziness, vertigo, and tingling or numbness (parasthesia) of the face, tongue, or extremities. Migraine without aura is the most prevalent type and may occur on one or both sides (bilateral) of the head. Tiredness or mood changes may be experienced the day before the headache. Nausea, vomiting, and sensitivity to light (photophobia) often accompany migraine without aura.

Abdominal migraine is most common in children with a family history of

migraine. Symptoms include abdominal pain without a gastrointestinal cause
(May last up to 72 hours), nausea, vomiting, and flushing or paleness (pallor).
Children who have abdominal migraine often develop typical migraine as
they age.

Basilar artery migraine involves a disturbance of the basilar artery in the
brainstem. Symptoms include severe headache, vertigo, double vision,
slurred speech, and poor muscle coordination. This type occurs primarily in
young people.

Carotidynia, also called lower-half headache or facial migraine, produces
deep, dull, aching, and sometimes piercing pain in the jaw or neck. There is
usually tenderness and swelling over the carotid artery in the neck. Episodes
can occur several times weekly and last a few minutes to hours. This type
occurs more commonly in older people. Doppler ultrasound studies of the
carotid arteries are normal.

Headache-free migraine is characterized by the presence of aura without
headache. This occurs in patients with a history of migraine with aura.

Ophthalmologic migraine begins with a headache felt in the eye and is
accompanied by vomiting. As the headache progresses, the eyelid droop
(ptosis) and nerves responsible for eye movement become paralyzed. Ptosis
may persist for days or weeks.

Status migraine is a rare type involving intense pain that usually lasts longer
than 72 hours. The patient may require hospitalization.

Incidence and Prevalence

Migraines afflict about 30 million people in the United States. They may
occur at any age, but usually begin between the ages of 10 and 40 and
diminish after age 50. Some people experience several migraines a month,
while others have only a few migraines throughout their lifetime.
Approximately 75% of migraine sufferers are women.

PREVENTION

Understanding your headache triggers can help you avoid foods and
situations that cause your migraines. Keep a headache diary to help identify
the source or trigger of your symptoms. Then modify your environment or
habits to avoid future headaches.

Other tips for preventing migraines include:

- Avoid smoking

- Avoid alcohol

- Avoid artificial sweeteners and other known food-related triggers

- Get regular exercise

- Get plenty of sleep each night

- Learn to relax and reduce stress -- some patients have found that biofeedback and self-hypnosis helps reduce the number of migraine attacks.

CLUSTER HEADACHE

A cluster headache is one-sided head pain that may involve tearing of the eyes and a stuffy nose. Attacks occur regularly for 1 week to 1 year, separated by long pain-free periods that last at least 1 month, possibly longer.

CAUSES

Cluster headaches are a fairly common form of chronic, repeated headaches. They are more common in men than women. The headaches can occur at any age but are most common in adolescence and middle age. They tend to run in families.

Scientists do not know exactly what causes cluster headaches, but they appear to be related to the body's sudden release of histamine or serotonin.

The following may trigger cluster attacks:

- Alcohol and cigarette smoking

- High altitudes (trekking, air travel)

- Bright light (including sunlight)

- Exertion

- Heat (hot weather, hot baths)

- Foods high in nitrites (such as bacon and preserved meats)

- Certain medications (including nitro-glycerine and various blood pressure medications)

- Cocaine

SYMPTOMS

A cluster headache begins as a severe, sudden headache. The headache most commonly strikes 2 to 3 hours after falling asleep, usually during the dreaming (rapid eye movement, or REM) phase. However, the headache may occur while you are awake. The headache tends to occur at the same time of day.

The pain occurs on one side of the head. It may be described as:

*   Burning

*   Sharp

*   Steady

The pain may occur in, behind, and around one eye. It may:

*   Involve one side of the face from neck to temples

*   Quickly gets worse, peaking within 5 to 10 minutes

The strongest pain may last 30 minutes to 2 hours.

The eye and nose on the same side of the head pain may also be affected. Symptoms can include:

*   Swelling under or around the eye (may affect both eyes)

*   Excessive tearing

*   Red eye

*   Rhino rhea (running nose) or one-sided stuffy nose (same side as the head pain)

*   Red, flushed face

Cluster headaches may occur daily for months, alternating with periods without headaches (episodic), or they can recur for a year or more without stopping (chronic).

TESTS

Your health care provider can diagnosis this type of headache by performing a physical exam and asking questions about your symptoms and medical history.

If a physical exam is done during an attack, the exam will usually reveal Horner Syndrome   (one-sided eyelid drooping or a small pupil). These symptoms will not be present at other times. No other neurological changes will be seen.

Tests, such as an MRI of the head, may be needed to rule out other causes for the headaches.

Treatment

Treatment does not cure cluster headaches. The goal of treatment is to relieve symptoms. The headaches may go away on their own, or you may need treatment to prevent them.

Smoking, alcohol use, specific foods, and other factors that seem to trigger cluster headaches should be avoided. A headache diary can help you identify your headache triggers. When you get a headache, write down the day and time the pain began. The diary should include notes about what you ate and drank in the last 24 hours, how much you slept and when, and what was going on in your life immediately before the pain started. For example, were you under any unusual stress? Also include information about how long the headache lasted, and what made it stop.

Treatment for cluster headaches involves:

- Methods to treat the pain when it happens

- Medicines to prevent the headaches

Your doctor may recommend the following treatments for when the headaches occurs:

A combination of medicines may be needed to control headache symptoms. Because each person responds differently to medicine, your doctor may have you try several medications before deciding which works best for you. Painkillers do not usually relieve the pain from cluster headaches. Generally, they take too long to work.

PROGNOSIS

Cluster headaches are not life-threatening and usually cause no permanent structural changes. However, they are chronic and often painful enough to interfere with work or lifestyle. Occasionally, the pain may be so severe that some people may consider self harm.

Side effects of medications or surgery may be severe.

POSSIBLE COMPLICATIONS

- Headaches that interfere with daily activities

- Horner Syndrome

- Side effects of medications
- Complications due to surgery to treat the headaches, including:
  o Permanent muscle weakness in the face or head
  o Decreased sensation in parts of the face or head

PREVENTION

If prone to cluster headache, stop smoking. Alcohol use and any foods that are associated with cluster headache may need to be avoided. Medications may prevent cluster headaches in some cases.

MIXED TENSION MIGRAINE

Mixed tension migraine is a headache with features of both tension and migraine headaches.

CAUSES

Migraine headaches affect millions of people. Tension headaches are even more common, affecting about 40% of the population. People with mixed tension migraine have features of both types of headaches.
It is difficult to differentiate which symptoms are due to which type of headache. Women have mixed tension migraines more often than men.

Common triggers for these headaches are hormonal changes, dietary factors, environmental factors, stimulation, and stress. Examples include:

- Alcohol
- Bright light
- Food and food additives
- Missed or delayed meals
- Menstruation
- Odours
- Too much or too little sleep
- Use and withdrawal of certain drugs or medications

SYMPTOMS

- Headache on one or both sides

o   Throbbing pain

o   May feel dull, tight, or like a band around the head

o   Pain varies from mild to severe

o   May get worse with activity

o   May last 4 - 72 hours (in some people, the headaches may occur every day)

- Nausea or vomiting

- Sensitivity to light or sound

- Irritability

- Depression

- Sluggishness

- Numbness, tingling, weakness

- Neck pain

TESTS

Your doctor will perform a physical exam, including a detailed examination of your nervous system, and ask you about your symptoms and family history.

Tests that may be done include:

- CT or MRI of the head and neck

- Blood work

- Lumbar puncture (spinal tap)

TREATMENT

Certain things may cause your headaches. For example, some people get headaches after drinking alcohol or eating certain foods. These are called triggers. You should identify your specific triggers and avoid them as much as possible.

A headache diary can help you identify your headache triggers. When you get a headache, write down the day and time the pain began. The diary should include notes about what you ate and drank in the last 24 hours, how much you slept and when, and what was going on in your life immediately before the pain started. For example, were you under any unusual stress? Also include information about how long the headache lasted, and what made it stop.

Hot or cold showers or baths may relieve a headache for some people. It is important to follow a healthy lifestyle, get plenty of sleep, and to avoid stress as much as possible.

Over-the-counter medicines such as ibuprofen and acetaminophen may help. If your headaches are severe, your doctor may prescribe other medicines to relieve your pain and prevent further attacks.

PROGNOSIS

Avoiding triggers and taking the appropriate medicine can help manage headache symptoms in many people.

Possible Complications

Pain medications only relieve headache symptoms for a short period of time. After a while, they do not work as well or the help they provide does not last as long. Regular, overuse of pain medications can
lead to rebound headaches. Typically this occurs in people who take pain medications 3 or more times a week on a regular basis.

It's important to see a doctor if you have chronic headaches. In some cases, the headache may be a symptom of a more serious disorder.

PREVENTION

Tips for preventing headaches:

- Avoid triggers.
- Get enough sleep.
- Eat a proper diet.
- Exercise regularly.

Medicine may be needed to prevent headaches.

TENSION HEADACHE

A tension headache is pain or discomfort in the head, scalp, or neck, usually associated with muscle tightness in these areas.

CAUSES

Tension headaches are one of the most common forms of headaches. They may occur at any age, but are most common in adults and adolescents.

If a headache occurs two or more times a week for several months or longer, the condition is considered chronic. Chronic daily headaches can result from the under- or over-treatment of a primary headache. For example, patients who take pain medication more than 3 days a week on a regular basis can develop rebound headaches.

Tension headaches can occur when the patient also has a migraine.

Tension headaches occur when neck and scalp muscles become tense, or contract. The muscle contractions can be a response to stress, depression, a head injury, or anxiety.

Any activity that causes the head to be held in one position for a long time without moving can cause a headache. Such activities include typing or other computer work, fine work with the hands, and using a microscope. Sleeping in a cold room or sleeping with the neck in an abnormal position may also trigger a tension headache.

Other triggers of tension headaches include:

- Alcohol use
- Caffeine (too much or withdrawal)
- Colds and the flu
- Dental problems such as jaw clenching or teeth grinding
- Eye strain
- Excessive smoking
- Fatigue
- Nasal congestion
- Overexertion
- Sinus infection

Tension headaches are not associated with structural changes in the brain.

Symptoms

The headache pain may be described as:

- Dull, pressure-like (not throbbing)
- A tight band on the head
- All over (not just in one point or one side)

- Worse in the scalp, temples, or back of the neck, and possibly in the shoulders

The pain may occur as an isolated event, constantly, or daily. Pain may last for 30 minutes to 7 days. It may be triggered by or get worse with stress, fatigue, noise, or glare.

There may be difficulty sleeping. Tension headaches usually do not cause nausea or vomiting.

People with tension headaches tend to try relieving pain by massaging their scalp, temples, or the bottom of the neck.

TESTS

A headache that is mild to moderate, not accompanied by other symptoms, and responds to home treatment within a few hours may not need further examination or testing, especially if it has occurred in

the past. A tension headache reveals no abnormal findings on a neurological exam. However, tender points (trigger points) in the muscles are often seen in the neck and shoulder areas.

The health care provider should be consulted -- to rule out other disorders that can cause headache -- if the headache is severe, persistent (does not go away), or if other symptoms are present with the headache.

Headaches that disturb sleep occur whenever you are active, or that are recurrent or chronic may require examination and treatment by a health care provider.

TREATMENT

Understanding your headache triggers can help you avoid situations that cause your headaches. A headache diary can help you identify your headache triggers. When you get a headache, write down the day and time the pain began. The diary should include notes about what you ate and drank in the last 24 hours, how much you slept and when, and what was going on in your life immediately before the pain started. For example, were you under any unusual stress? Also include information about how long the headache lasted, and what made it stop.

Hot or cold showers or baths may relieve a headache for some people. You may need to make lifestyle changes if you have chronic tension headaches. This may include changing your sleep habits (usually to get more sleep), increasing exercise, and stretching the neck and back muscles. In some situations, you may need to change your job or recreational habits.

Over-the-counter painkillers such as aspirin, ibuprofen, or acetaminophen may relieve pain if relaxation techniques do not work. If you are planning to take part in an activity that you know will trigger a headache, taking one of these painkillers beforehand may be helpful.

Narcotic pain relievers are sometimes prescribed. Remember that pain medications only relieve headache symptoms for a short period of time. After a while, they do not work as well or the help they provide does not last as long. Regular, overuse of pain medications can lead to rebound headaches.

Combining drug treatment with relaxation or stress-management training, biofeedback, cognitive behavioural therapy, or acupuncture may provide better relief for chronic headaches.

Botox (botulinum toxin) is becoming popular as a treatment for chronic daily headaches, including tension headaches. However, it is currently not approved for such use.

PROGNOSIS

Tension headaches usually respond well to treatment without residual effects.

Although they are not medically dangerous, chronic tension headaches can have a negative impact on the quality of life and work productivity.

Possible Complications

Rebound headaches -- headaches that keep coming back -- may occur from overuse of painkillers.

It's important to see a doctor if you have chronic headaches. In some cases, the headache may be a symptom of a more serious disorder.

PREVENTION

Learn and practice stress management. Some people find relaxation exercises or meditation helpful. Biofeedback may improve relaxation exercises and may be helpful for chronic tension headache.

Tips to prevent tension headaches:

- Keep warm if the headache is associated with cold.
- Use a different pillow or change sleeping positions.
- Practice good posture when reading, working, or doing other

activities.

•   Exercise the neck and shoulders frequently when typing, working on computers, or doing other close work.

•   Get plenty of sleep and rest.

.   Massaging sore muscles may also help.

STRESS MANAGEMENT

Stress is a feeling of emotional or physical tension.

Emotional stress usually occurs in situations people consider difficult or challenging. Different people consider different situations to be stressful.

Physical stress refers to a physical reaction of the body to various triggers. The pain experienced after surgery is an example of physical stress. Physical stress often leads to emotional stress, and emotional stress often occurs as physical stress (e.g., stomach cramps).

Stress management involves controlling and reducing the tension that occurs in stressful situations by making emotional and physical changes. The degree of stress and the desire to make the changes will determine how much change takes place.

ASSESSING STRESS

Attitude: A person's attitude can influence whether or not a situation or emotion is stressful. A person with a negative attitude will often report more stress than would someone with a positive attitude.

Diet: A poor diet puts the body in a state of physical stress and weakens the immune system. As a result, a person can be more likely to get infections. A poor diet can mean unhealthy food choices, not eating enough, or not eating on a normal schedule.

This form of physical stress also decreases the ability to deal with emotional stress, because not getting the right nutrition may affect the way the brain processes information.

Physical activity: Not getting enough physical activity can put the body in a stressed state. Physical activity has many benefits, including promoting a feeling of well-being.

Support systems: Almost everyone needs someone in their life they can rely on when they are having a hard time. Having little or no support makes stressful situations even more difficult to deal with.

Relaxation: People with no outside interests, hobbies, or other ways to relax may be less able to handle stressful situations.

AN INDIVIDUAL STRESS MANAGEMENT PROGRAM

- Find the positive in situations, and don't dwell on the negative.
- Plan fun activities
- Take regular breaks.

Physical activity:

- Start a physical activity program. Most experts recommend 20 minutes of aerobic activity three times per week.
- Decide on a specific type, amount, and level of physical activity. Fit this into your schedule so it can be part of your routine.
- Find a buddy to exercise with -- it is more fun and it will encourage you to stick with your routine.
- You do not have to join a gym -- 20 minutes of brisk walking outdoors is enough.

Nutrition:

- Eat foods that improve your health and well-being. For example, increase the amount of fruits and vegetables you eat.
- Use the food guide pyramid to help you make healthy food choices.
- Eat normal-sized portions on a regular schedule.

Social support:

- Make an effort to socialize. Even though you may feel tempted to avoid people when you feel stressed, meeting friends usually helps people feel less stressed.
- Be good to yourself and others.

Relaxation:

•	Learn about and try using relaxation techniques, such as guided imagery, listening to music, or practicing yoga or meditation. With some practice, these techniques should work for you.

•	Listen to your body when it tells you to slow down or take a break.

•	Make sure to get enough sleep. Good sleep habits are one of the best ways to manage stress.

•	Take time for personal interests and hobbies.

RESOURCES

If these stress management techniques do not work for you, there are professionals, such as licensed social workers, psychologists, and psychiatrists, who can help. Schedule time with one of these mental health professionals to help you learn stress management strategies, including relaxation techniques. Support groups of various types are also available in most communities. You can consult an experienced homoeopathic physician.

CHILDREN AND HEADACHE

Headaches are common in children. Headaches that begin early in life can develop into migraines as the child grows older. Migraines in children or adolescents can develop into tension-type headaches at any

time. In contrast to adults with migraine, young children often feel migraine pain on both sides of the head and have headaches that usually last less than 2 hours. Children may look pale and appear restless

or irritable before and during an attack. Other children may become nauseous, lose their appetite, or feel pain elsewhere in the body during the headache.

Headaches in children can be caused by a number of triggers, including emotional problems such as tension between family members, stress from school activities, weather changes, irregular eating and sleep,

dehydration, and certain foods and drinks. Of special concern among children are headaches that occur after head injury or those accompanied by rash, fever, or sleepiness.

It may be difficult to identify the type of headache because children often have problems describing where it hurts, how often the headaches occur, and how long they last. Asking a child with a headache to

draw a picture of where the pain is and how it feels can make it easier for the doctor to determine the proper treatment.

Migraine in particular is often misdiagnosed in children. Parents and caretakers sometimes have to be detectives to help determine that a child has migraine. Clues to watch for include sensitivity to light and

noise, which may be suspected when a child refuses to watch television or use the computer, or when the child stops playing to lie down in a dark room. Observe whether or not a child is able to eat during a

headache. Very young children may seem cranky or irritable and complain of abdominal pain (abdominal migraine).

Headache treatment in children and teens usually includes rest, fluids, and over-the-counter pain relief medicines. Always consult with a physician before giving headache medicines to a child. Most tension-type headaches in children can be treated with over-the-counter medicines that are marked for children with usage guidelines based on the child's age and weight. Headaches in some children may also be treated effectively using relaxation/behavioral therapy. Children with cluster headache may be treated with oxygen therapy early in the initial phase of the attacks.

Headache and Sleep Disorders

Headaches are often a secondary symptom of a sleep disorder. For example, tension-type headache is regularly seen in persons with insomnia or sleep-wake cycle disorders. Nearly three-fourths of individuals who suffer from narcolepsy complain of either migraine or cluster headache. Migraines and cluster headaches appear to be related to the number of and transition between rapid eye movement (REM) and other sleep periods an individual has during sleep. Hypnic headache awakens individuals mainly at night but may also interrupt daytime naps. Reduced oxygen levels in people with sleep apnoea may trigger early morning headaches.

Getting the proper amount of sleep can ease headache pain. Generally, too little or too much sleep can worsen headaches, as can overuse of sleep medicines. Daytime naps often reduce deep sleep at night and can produce headaches in some adults. Some sleep disorders and secondary headache are treated using antidepressants. Check with a doctor before using over the-counter medicines to ease sleep-associated headaches.

Coping with Headache

Headache treatment is a partnership between you and your doctor, and honest communication is essential. Finding a quick fix to your headache may not be possible. It may take some time for your doctor or specialist to determine the best course of treatment. Avoid using over-the-counter medicines more than twice a week, as they may actually worsen headache pain and the frequency of attacks. Visit a local headache support group meeting (if available) to learn how others with headache cope with their pain and discomfort. Relax whenever possible to ease stress and related symptoms, get enough sleep, regularly perform aerobic exercises, and eat a regularly scheduled and healthy diet that avoids food triggers. Gaining more control over your headache, stress, and emotions will make you feel better and let you embrace daily activities as much as possible.

HOMOEOPATHIC TREATMENT for MIGRAINE and Other HEADACHES

Homoeopathy is based on symptom similarity and totality of symptoms. Chief medicines include Belladona, Natrum Mur, Iris Versicolor, Sanguinaria, Spigelia, Bryonia, Nux Vomica etc. Medicines may differ from person to person.

For a right medicine you should consult a qualified homoeopathic practitioner or can consult me on ***drs108@gmail.com***. Certainly, you have to pay my fee.

AYURVEDIC TREATMENT OF MIGRAINE

Migraine has become a common disorder owing to modern lifestyle. From the perspective of ayurveda, migraine headaches are due to a disorder in tridosha - the mind-body constitution. Although it is possible to get headaches from disorders in vata, pitta, or kapha, migraines frequently occur when systemic pitta moves into the cardiovascular system, circulates, and affects the blood vessels around the brain. The blood vessels dilate due to the hot, sharp quality of pitta. This, in turn, creates pressure on the nerves, resulting in migraines. Pitta disorders are characterized by the red complexion and eyes, light sensitivity, burning sensation, anger, irritability, and nose bleeds. So, the treatment involves following the recommendations for pitta pacifying foods, herbs and lifestyle.

Avoid hot, spicy foods, fermented foods, and sour or citrus fruits. A pitta-soothing diet is effective both for migraine relief and as a preventive measure.

Preventive Breakfast

If you are one of those individuals who get migraines at midday, which then subside later in the evening, there is a preventive approach available from ayurveda. It is simple, but effective.

First thing in the morning, take 1 ripe banana. Peel it, chop it into pieces, and add 1 teaspoon warm ghee, 1 teaspoon date sugar, and a pinch of cardamom on top. This is delicious, and it will help to reduce pitta and prevent a headache from arising.

Herbal Remedy

The following herbal compound is beneficial in managing migraine-

Shatavari 5 parts

Brahmi 4 parts

Jatamamsi 3 parts

Mukta 3 parts

Prepare this mixture, and take 1/2 teaspoon twice a day, morning and evening, after breakfast and dinner, with a little lukewarm water. This formula is designed to pacify the aggravated pitta and help relieve migraine headaches.

Purgatives (such as aloe vera gel, rhubarb, and fennel), liver cleansers (such as amalaki and brahmi), sandalwood oil on the third eye, temples, heart, and under the nose, medicated oils or ghee, using gudachi, bala, and ashwagandha; fomentation, and saturating snuff are also advised.

Long-term healing includes chyavanprash, brahmi, and ashwagandha.

Migraines from Vata Imbalance:

As mentioned migraines can also originate due to imbalance in vata dosha. The symptoms of vata imbalance are: anxiety, depression, dry skin, constipation and extreme pain. The recommended treatment is: triphala as a purgative, jatamanshi, brahmi and rest. Shiro dhara (hot oil head massage) is also recommended.

Migraines from Kapha Imbalance:

This condition is characterized by dull headache, heaviness, fatigue, nausea, white or clear phlegm, vomiting, and excess salivation. Respiratory disorders are often associated with these symptoms. The recommended treatment is: trikatu, brahmi, Tulsa tea, inhaling eucalyptus oil, and nasal snuff of ginger or pepper. Shiro dhara (hot oil head massage) is also recommended.

Suvarna Sutashekhara

This is the most commonly prescribed Ayurvedic drug for treating migraine. It is not just a preventive but also a curative means.

Ingredients: Many items are used to prepare this medication. These elements are borax and sulphur in the 'bhasma' form, sulphur, copper, gold and mercury.

Moreover, 10 medicinal plants and drugs (extracted from animal sources) are added to the mixture.

Besides, two other strong drugs (which are poisonous in their raw forms) – Dhatura and Vatsanabha – are processed to make them not only potent but also pure. After processing, these two drugs are made free from having any side effects on a patient.

All of these are mixed in definite ratios. To this mixture is added Bhringaraja juice.

Dose: It is given in the dose of 125 milligram twice daily. The medication is to be taken with milk.

Godanti Bhasma

This is a rather inexpensive but effective Ayurvedic medication for patients suffering from migraine.

Dose: It is given in the dose of one gram thrice daily. The medication is to be taken with honey.

Shadbindu Taila

This Ayurvedic medicated oil is quite effective in treating migraine. This medication irritates the nasal mucous membrane. However, it effects instant relief.

Ingredient: This drug is to be taken with mustard oil.

Dose: Only six drops are to be taken in each nostril daily and till the symptoms persist.

Anu Taila

Proper use of this oil brings about instant relief to acute and chronic migraine instances.

This medicated oil needs to be inhaled deeply to induce forced sneezing. It removes the nasal blockages from the sinuses and their passages. The nerves in the nasal routes are soothed.

Even as the mental strain is removed, the heaviness in the head is also relieved. The patient will be able to sleep soundly. Above all, there are no side effects.

Ingredients: It is prepared from 26 medicinal plants. The definite proportions of these plants are then boiled in goat's milk and gingerly oil.

Dose: One needs to drop at least 15 drops of this oil in each nostril to induce sneezing. This medicated oil needs to be inhaled at least thrice daily.

Panchakarma for Migraine and Headaches

Pre-purification therapies: Pre-purification therapies are the first ones applied to loosen the toxins, open up the circulation channels and get the body ready for discarding these wastes. These methods are highly relaxing for the body and mind.

The following pre-purification methods are usually adopted for treating Migraines and Headaches.

Shirodhara

In this process herbal oil, medicated milk, medicated butter milk etc, are poured on the forehead in a special method for about 45-50 minutes. Highly effective in providing both temporary and permanent relief from Migraines and Headaches. Ingredients used in Sirodhara include gooseberry, sandalwood...

Thakradhara

This treatment involves continuous pouring of medicated buttermilk on the forehead. It cools the head and gives immediate relief from headaches. It also has a soothing effect on the eyes.

Omelettes, nut grass tuber and staff tree are the medicinal herbs used.

Thalami Special powder mixed with medicated oil is applied on head vertex and retained for 20 to 45 minutes. Medicinal herbs used are Sida plant Indian Penny worth and the Staff tree.

OTHER TREATMENTS

There are certain other preventions and treatments for migraine, cluster headaches and other types of headache-

Avoid Direct Sun

Because migraine headaches are predominantly a pitta disorder, they are affected by the hot sun. When the sun rises, it's hot, sharp, penetrating rays increase pitta in the cardiovascular system and cause the dilation of the blood vessels in the brain, which results in the painful headaches. So avoid direct exposure to the sun. If you have to go out, use an umbrella or wear a hat or other protection from the sun.

One should avoid direct exposure of cold too.

Nature walks

Walks in the full moon and by water; and flower gardening reduce Pitta causes of migraines.

Soothing Nose Drops

Once a headache has developed, putting about 5 drops of warm brahmi ghee in each nostril will help relieve the pain.

Head Massage

Shirodhara (hot oil head massage) is also beneficial.

Recommended Yoga Postures

Moon Salutation is especially good for migraines. Yoga postures such as the Hidden Lotus, Boat pose, Bow pose, Spinal Twist, Palm Tree pose, and

Standing on the Toes are also good to combat migraines.

A Cooling Pranayama

Do a cooling breathing exercise such as shitali. To do it, curl your tongue into a tube. Inhale slowly through the curled tongue, swallow, and then exhale normally through the nose, keeping the mouth closed.

You will feel the incoming air cool your saliva, your tongue and the oral mucous membranes.

This breathing exercise will lower the body temperature, and make the saliva cool. It also helps to quench thirst, and improves digestion, absorption and assimilation.

If you can't curl your tongue into a tube, an alternative way to perform shitali is with your teeth lightly clenched together and your tongue pressed up against the teeth. The air is then inhaled through the teeth.

Some people feel pain when coot air is drawn through the teeth; keeping your tongue against your teeth will provide warmth and prevent this discomfort.

A Healing Yawn

When you have a migraine, gently squeeze your earlobes, pulling the ear down, and do the act of yawning. This will relieve the pressure on the blood vessels and help to pacify the headache.

Avoid overexertion.

HOME TREATMENT OF MIGRAINE

Wet a towel, squeeze it and keep it in the freezer for around 5 – 7 minutes. Now, take the frozen towel and keep it over your head and eyes. You will notice immediate relief from the severe pain. Another highly effective alternative is to opt for a good head/scalp massage. Lie down in a room that is dark and peaceful and without any environmental disturbances. Allow a massage expert to gently apply flowing strokes to your head and scalp to bring you relief from the pain. In the absence of a massage therapist, you may try massaging the head yourself. This can be done by massaging the scalp and head by rubbing the aching areas in gentle circular motions.

Aromatherapy

Aromatherapy has been found to be quite effective in relieving the painful symptoms of a migraine attack. In aromatherapy, the most regularly used essential oils used for providing relief from migraine attacks include lavender and peppermint. These essential oils are helpful in easing stress, tensions and migraines. Do bear in mind that not all individuals find relief from using aromatherapy. Ginger is one of the most effective solutions to ease pain caused during migraine attacks. It has a high content of anti inflammatory properties, which are beneficial in promoting blood circulation and relaxing the blood Vessels. The consumption of fresh ginger or powdered ginger in a slightly cooked form can also prove to be advantageous in obtaining relief from pain caused due to migraine attack.

Always remember to drink lots of water. Keeping one's self well hydrated is believed to be one of the most effective home remedies for migraine attacks. There are many cases where headaches can begin due to severe dehydration and thus it is extremely critical to ensure that you drink sufficient amounts of water. Ideally, it is recommended that you drink about a liter of water daily.

Identify the reasons which are triggering your attacks. There are different triggers for different individuals. Some individuals are affected by a particular food where as others are affected by excessive stress.

Determining your specific triggers will help you in preventing migraine attacks in the future.

Once used to treat a variety of conditions, including headaches and fever, feverfew has been "rediscovered" by migraine sufferers, who are using the herb to blunt the sometimes crippling pain that accompanies their sudden and ill-understood attacks.

Scientists now know that feverfew contains chemicals that may prevent migraines. And the best news is that feverfew has few side effects.

Some people get some relief by applying either a cold or warm compress to the affected area. Most people report that a cold compress works best, but if that is not effective, try a warm compress.

Acupressure

Acupressure is also one of the good home remedies for migraine headaches. Like acupuncture, it is a well-known alternative treatment for many medical problems that has been used for thousands of years.

To get headache pain relief, squeeze the fleshy area between your thumb and forefinger for at least five minutes for one of the quick remedies for migraines. Many folks also can relieve migraine pain by gently rubbing using small circular motions.

TIPS TO CONTROL HEADACHES

Try the following tips for your occasional headache pain. If you're headaches are frequent or severe, be sure to discuss them with a medical professional.

Try -- but don't overdo -- pain pills. A dose of an over-the-counter (OTC) analgesic, such as aspirin, acetaminophen, or ibuprofen, is often enough to alleviate the occasional headache. But if you take more than two doses a day frequently or for more than four or five days in a row to relieve headache pain, contact your doctor. Taking pain relievers too often can actually worsen your headache pain. For a list of precautions to take when using over-the-counter analgesics,

Lie down. Lying down and closing your eyes for half an hour or more may be one of the best treatments for a bad headache. For some types of headaches, such as migraines, sleep is the only thing that seems to interrupt the pain cycle. Recognizing the early signs of a headache can keep the pain from getting out of control, since doctors say the sooner you get to bed or lie on a sofa, the sooner a headache will fade.

Don't let the sun shine in. Especially if your symptoms resemble those of a migraine (such as severe pain on one side of the head, nausea, blurred vision, and extreme sensitivity to light), resting in a darkened room may alleviate the pain, experts agree. Bright light may also cause headaches. Even staring at a glowing computer screen may be enough to trigger pain on the brain. Wearing tinted glasses or using other means to filter bright light and minimize glare may help prevent headaches.

Use a cold compress. A washcloth dipped in ice-cold water and placed over the eyes or an ice pack placed on the site of the pain is other good ways of relieving a headache. You might also see if your pharmacy sells special ice packs that surround the whole head (known as "headache hats") or frozen gel-packs that can be inserted into pillows. Whatever you use, keep in mind that speed is critical: Using ice as soon as possible after the onset of the headache will relieve the pain within 20 minutes for most people.

Try heat if ice feels uncomfortable to you, or if it doesn't help your headache, try placing a warm washcloth over your eyes or on the site of the pain. Leave the compress on for half an hour, re-warming it as necessary.

Think pleasant thoughts many headaches are brought on or worsened by stress and tension. Learning to handle life's difficulties by tuning out unpleasant thoughts may keep the volume down on a bad headache. When you feel your body shifting into crisis mode after you have a serious disagreement with a spouse or co-worker, for example -- force yourself to think pleasant thoughts. Relaxing your mind will help you figure out a way to resolve the problem, which can help ward off headache-causing tension.

Check for tension Along with the preceding tip, stop periodically during the day and check your body for tension. Are you clenching your jaw or wrinkling your brow? Are your hands balled-up into fists? If you discover these signs of tension, stop, relax, and take a deep breath or two (don't go beyond a couple of deep breaths, though, otherwise you may begin to hyperventilate). Occasional body checks like this could nip a headache in the bud.

Quit Smoking- Smoking may bring on or worsen a headache, especially if you suffer from cluster headaches -- extremely painful headaches that last from 5 to 20 minutes and come in groups.

Don't drink Drinking more alcohol than you're used to often causes a notorious morning-after effect -- a pounding headache. But even a single serving of some alcoholic beverages can trigger headaches, including the migraine and cluster varieties, in certain people. For example, dark alcoholic beverages such as red wines, sherry, brandy, scotch, vermouth, and beer contain large amounts of tyramine, an amino acid that can spark headaches in people who are sensitive to it. And some people appear to be sensitive to the histamine in beer and wine. So if you're struggling with headaches, abstaining may be your best choice.

Start a program of regular exercise Regular exercise helps release the physical and emotional tension that may lead to headaches. Walking, jogging, and other aerobic activities help boost the body's production of endorphins (natural pain-relieving substances).

Cut down on caffeine the same chemical in coffee and tea that perks you up in the morning can also make your muscles tense and send your anxiety level through the roof. Consuming too much caffeine can also cause insomnia, which can trigger headaches. Another problem is that many people drink several cups of coffee a day during their work week but cut their consumption on Saturdays and Sundays. This pattern can lead to weekend caffeine-withdrawal headaches.

If caffeine is giving you a headache, wean yourself off the stimulating stuff by cutting your intake slowly. Start by eliminating the equivalent of one-half cup coffee per week until you are only drinking one cup of caffeinated coffee (or its equivalent) per day. One five-ounce cup of drip coffee contains about 150 milligrams of caffeine. A five-ounce cup of tea brewed for three to five minutes may contain 20 to 50 milligrams of caffeine. And cola drinks contain about 35 to 45 milligrams of caffeine per 12-ounce serving. Look out for stealth sources of caffeine, too, particularly in the OTC drugs in your medicine cabinet.

Fight the nausea first Some headaches may be accompanied by nausea, which can make you feel even worse. What's more, the gastric juices produced by stomach upset may hinder the absorption of certain prescription and OTC analgesics, which may make these drugs less effective at relieving the pain of your headache. So by first taking care of the nausea, the pain of the headache may be easier to treat. Many patients find that drinking peach juice, apricot nectar, or flat cola helps alleviate nausea. Anti nauseates may also be useful.

Rise and retire at the same time every day Oversleeping can create changes in body chemistry that set off migraines and other headaches. Going to bed and getting up at the same time every day -- including weekends -- keeps your body in a stable rhythm.

Keep a headache diary. If you get frequent headaches, try to tease out the factors that seem to be responsible. Get a notebook and keep track of your headaches. Rate each one on a scale of 0 to 3, starting with no headache (a score of 0) and moving up in intensity to mild headache (a score of 1), moderate to severe headache (a score of 2), and incapacitating headache (a score of 3). Record details about potential headache triggers. Were you under an unusual amount of stress? What did you eat? If you're a woman, did you have your period? Did you use medications that contain hormones, such as oral contraceptives? Now look for patterns by connecting days when you had bad headaches with these factors. This information may help you avoid triggers and can also help your physician devise a better treatment plan.

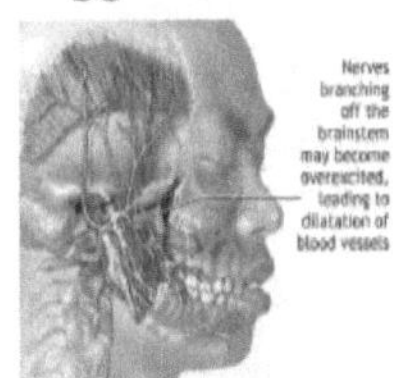

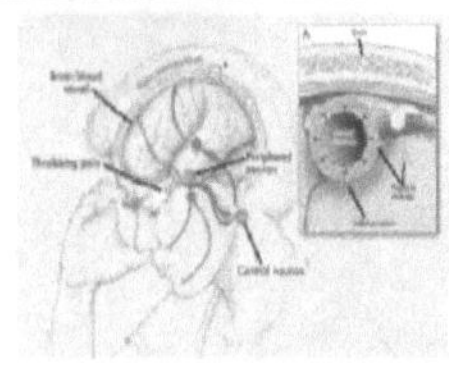

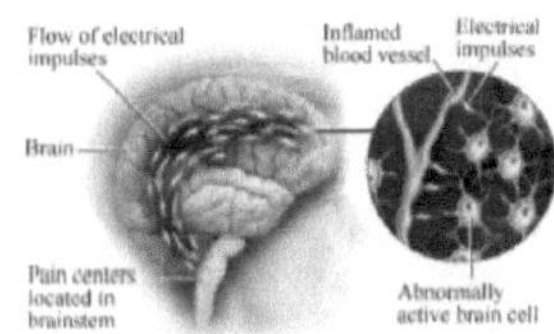

www.ingramcontent.com/pod-product-compliance
Lightning Source LLC
Chambersburg PA
CBHW020947160726
47993CB00007B/2979